Dear Bill,

It's Thursday which means I am writing to tell you I love you. Not much has happened today. I walked the dogs and did some laundry. I worked on some spreadsheets and in a moment, I will be cooking you some enchiladas. This morning at the gym, I swam 2000 yards and then sat in the hot tub for a while thinking about how great it is to be alive even when life is hard. I hope your day was happy. See you soon.

xo,

DS

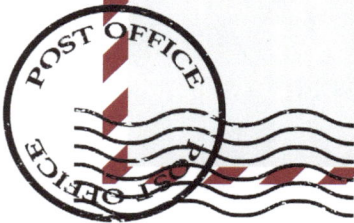

I began going on chemo dates at the age of 33 when my husband was going through chemo and we were forced into the lovely world of cancer. We had a five-year-old and three-year-old at home and we were at the hospital a lot. Their grandma took care of them for us.

Chemo for Bill was four days in a row every 21 days. We spent many long hours in the infusion center. He had a private room with a bed and television and a recliner for me to sit on. I almost never sat on the recliner.

I hopped onto the bed with him (a tiny twin bed or gurney) and wrapped myself up in his warm, cozy blankets.

It was 2003, so you have to understand that technology was good then, but not like today. We carried a tiny portable DVD player with us and I would grab snacks and a latte (I was always cold) and if he could tolerate food, he would order from the patient menu.

One night as we sat there in that bed with our movies and snacks, I turned to him (while poison was pumping through his veins of course) and said, "wow, this is great. We have free babysitting and all we have to do for the next several days is lay here in a bed and watch movies and eat. It's a guaranteed date every three weeks!"

We laughed. It was funny because it was true. The nurses loved us. They always made comments about how happy we seemed and how they really liked walking into our room.

Statistically, most marriages that include a life-threatening illness end in divorce. Deciding that chemo dates were fun was just one of millions of ways we fought cancer and kept our marriage strong.

This book is filled with activities you and your spouse can do together. Even if your spouse doesn't have cancer, there will be times of sickness, but fun and laughter can always happen. In fact, these date activities can be done when y'all are super healthy!

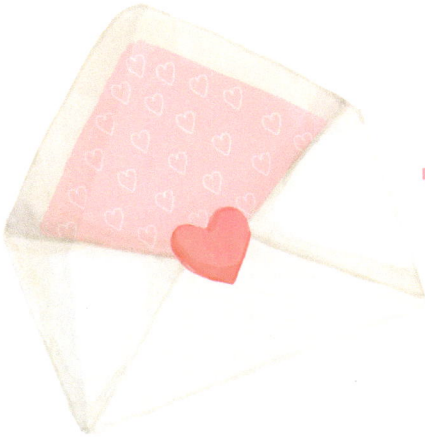

THURSDAY LETTERS

ACTIVITY: Write each other letters!

Not long after my husband Bill and I got married, we started writing each other a letter every Thursday. Before bed, we would exchange letters and somehow, it made us go to sleep happy even during difficult times.

Although our letters started out mostly hand-written, over the years, they turned into many different types of "letters". Sometimes they were funny. Sometimes they were romantic. Sometimes they were several pages long while other times, they might just be one or two lines.

Fun Thursday Letters

ways to write, sing or illustrate a love letter

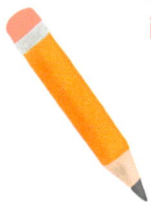

a hand-written note is so romantic these days

write a poem or song (and take it a step further by singing it)

For one of my Thursday letters, I wrote an entire "book{" for Bill called the "Bill Book" and it was filled with funny stories, recipes, jokes and not-very-well-done illustrations because I am not an artist.

scavenger hunt — yes, I have done this a couple of times. He comes home and has to search all over the house for clues until he finally finds his letter

special gift — sometimes he and I will give each other a sweet gift as a letter such as a pretty plant or a photo or chocolate or jewelry or a bottle of wine with a note attached

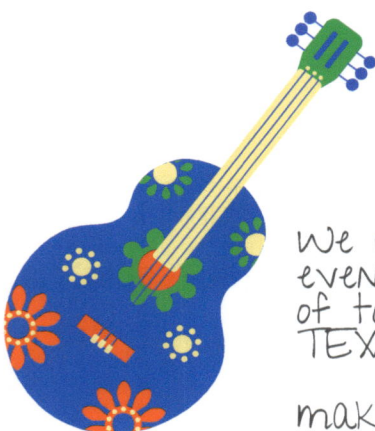

I speak Spanish, but Bill does not, so sometimes I write my letters in Spanish and make him figure out what they say!

We don't skip Thursday letters even if we are apart. Being out of town just means EMAIL or TEXT or even better...

making a funny video

There are millions of books out there about love and marriage. Marriage is hard. It requires constant work, so if you are considering marriage, just know that even though it's fun and wonderful, it never stops being hard work. If you don't like to work hard, don't get married.

Choose L♥VE even when you don't feel like it.

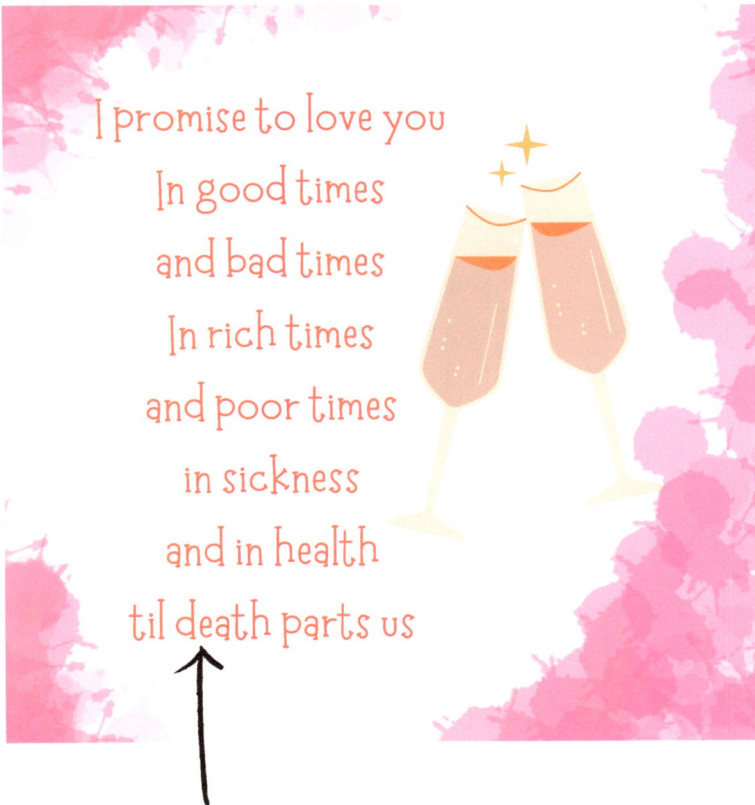

I promise to love you
In good times
and bad times
In rich times
and poor times
in sickness
and in health
til death parts us

That is a pretty big oath to make!

love

love
/ləv/
noun
an intense feeling of deep affection
verb
to feel deep affection for someone

here are some synonyms for love:

fondness

enchantment

affection

devotion

tenderness

delight

adoration

passion

allegiance

like

zeal

attachment

enamored

partiality

appreciation

But all those are just words. They are pretty words. but loving someone with just words only goes so far. It is nice to hear those words. BUT...

Real love is not what we say. Real love is what we do.

WAYS TO LOVE SOMEONE

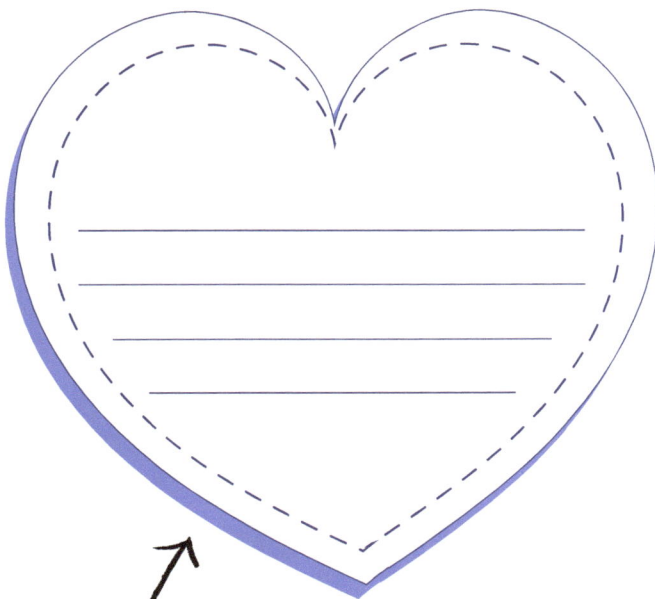

First, write a few ways you like to BE LOVED

Before you start thinking this is a book about love languages... nope. Go buy that book because it is really cool to figure out your own love language and then to know your husband's love language (and kids and friends, etc).

Instead, this book is more of a guide for those who need actual practical help loving someone during chemo and not only that, but this book has all kinds of activities for y'all to do together whether you're in the chemo unit or in the hospital or at home when you're just not feeling all that great. So, it's not just for cancer patients because let's face it... sometimes people get sick or have a surgery or a pandemic happens and you're on lockdown.

Keep "dating" and having fun together!

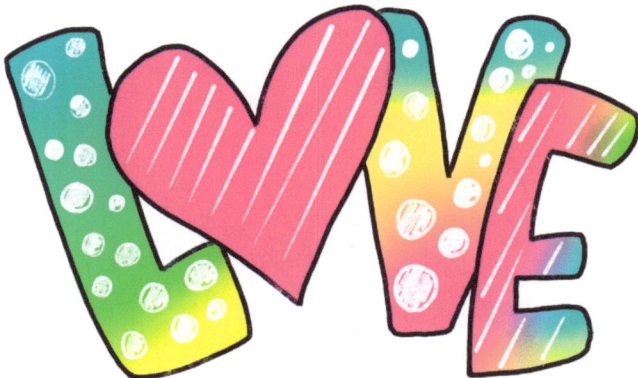

💜 Sitting on a blanket looking at the stars

🧡 Dancing in the kitchen

💛 Sipping wine by a fire pit

ways to love each other
that don't cost a thing

❤️ Hiking together in the mountains

💙 Swimming laps together

💜 Walking the dogs through the neighborhood

🧡 Cooking a pot of chili together

💛 Volunteering together

❤️ Playing board games

💙 Holding hands while you binge watch a show

When I was in college, some of my girlfriends and I were up late talking about what we wanted in a future husband. We said all kinds of things which I'm sure were unrealistic, but it was fun anyway. One of the things I said was...

I will know that I have found "the one" because I will come home to my apartment one day to find it full of balloons

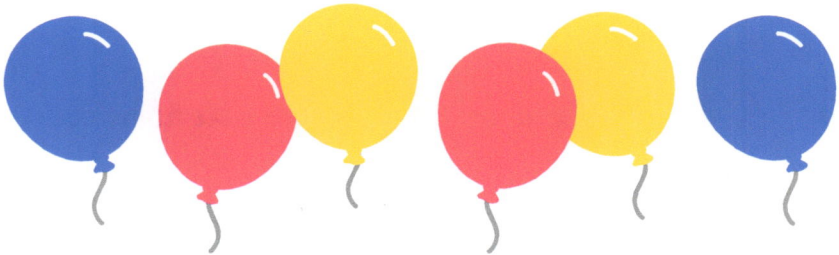

I was about 18 years old when I made that statement and forgot about it by the next day. So, fast forward... I am in my 20s and I am engaged to Bill. I am a teacher and it's Valentine's Day and my co-worker is getting married after work. I have promised her that I will get all of her gifts to her place after the ceremony and take care of her dog and I am also running late for work. So, my Friday morning is rushed.

I grab my coffee and my huge bag for work and head out the door. As I approach my car, I see it is full of balloons. Huge balloons with hearts all over them. In the front and in the back. In fact, the car is so full, I can't get in it.

You see, even though Bill hates staying up late and in those days, I always stayed up til at least 11:30 p.m., he had waited outside of my apartment til my lights were out and blew up 200 balloons to fill up my car. He didn't get to bed til probably 1:00 in the morning! Y'all, that is LOVE.

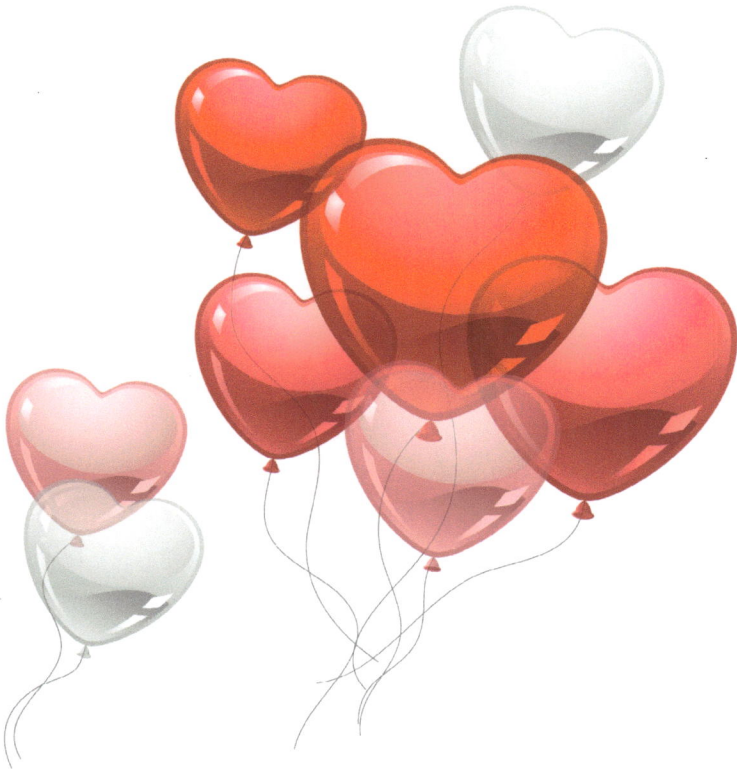

I was late for work. I was stressed about the day. But there I stood, getting as many balloons out of my car as I needed to so I could drive, with tears in my eyes. I found the man of my dreams. Someone willing to sacrifice his need to sleep so he could do something that would make my heart happy.

He had no idea that I had ever fantasized about a home full of balloons. I had forgotten myself until that moment. Real love.

Y'all, DO those kinds of things even after you're married. Don't ever stop being girlfriend and boyfriend!

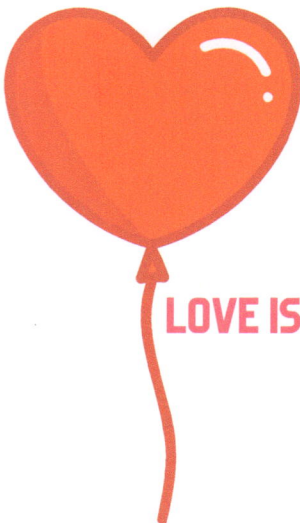

LOVE IS WHAT WE DO FOR OTHERS

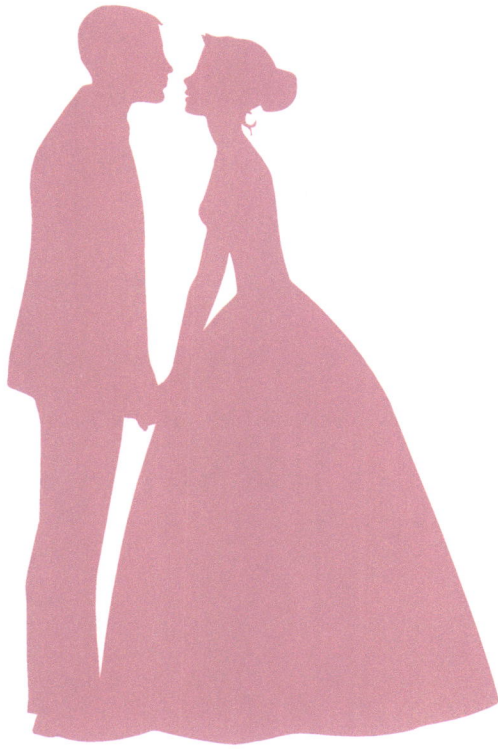

Let's go back to those vows for a moment. You said you would love each other in the **good** times and in the **rich** times and in the **healthy** times. It is so much fun and it is so easy in those times!

But you also said you would love each other in the **bad** times and the **poor** times and the **sick** times and truth be told, when one of you gets cancer, you could be facing bad, poor and sick all at once. That is no fun and it is absolutely not easy.

So, one of you is sick. Y'all can't go out on fun dates like you did when you were young and first dating. Can you have fun? YES! These next pages are filled with activities, humor, stories to share and so much more. So grab a pencil or two, pour a cup of something warm, snuggle under that blanket together and let's have fun on our CHEMO DATE!

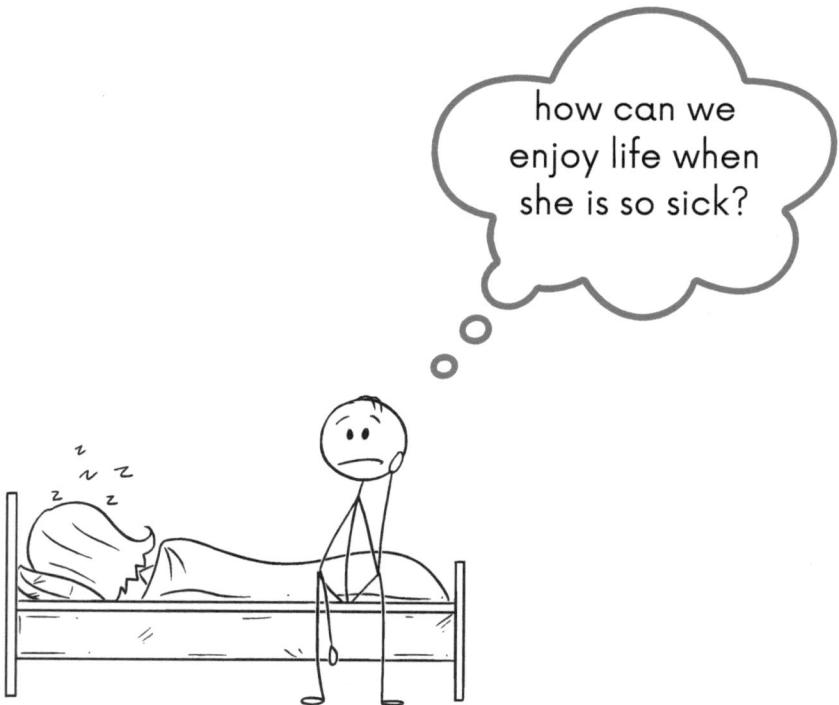

how can we enjoy life when she is so sick?

LIST FOR CHEMO DATE

- [ ] This book
- [ ] Blanket (in case they don't have one you like in the hospital)
- [ ] Candy and snacks
- [ ] laptop with a good streaming service to watch movies
- [ ] super comfy socks to keep your feet warm
- [ ] super cool playlist of your favorite songs
- [ ] books and magazines
- [ ] deck of cards
- [ ] board games
- [ ] phone with an updated podcast app
- [ ] small arts and craft kit

activity:

TOP TEN LIST

A long time ago, there was a late night television show host who did some really funny top ten lists. When Bill was going through chemo, he and I used to make our own top ten lists in the waiting rooms all the time. Here are some examples from our own life, but trust me, you gotta try making your own to keep yourself entertained.

Top Ten Barium Flavors
10. Chalk (not sure really)
9. Plain
8. Banana
7. Berry
6. Vanilla (we think)
5. Strawberry
4. Peach?
3. Some kind of cream
2. Chocolate
1. "Margarita" (no idea why)

Side note... we got very creative and came up with the concept of the Barium Bar. There would be a bartender serving up great barium cocktails and there would be body shots and music. I mean, if you gotta gulp down three huge cups full of this nastiness, why not make it fun?

Top Ten Names Bill Has Been Called by the Nurses

10. Lance Armstrong
9. Sweetie
8. 570018
7. "The Young Man With A Whole Lot of Cancer" (ouch!)
6. Will
5. Crew
4. Mr. Williams
3. Cruz (read about this below)
2. Mr. Crow
1. J.R. (you must read this one on the next page!)

"Cruz" was one of those interesting moments. The nurse walks out and says "Cruz" and we thought she was saying "Crews", so we got up. No one else got up. She checked his medical bracelet and asked him for his patient ID. She weighed him and took his blood pressure and escorted us to his room. I sat on the recliner by his bed while he jumped into the bed. Soon, another nurse walked in with a puzzled look on her face and asked, "which one of you is the patient?"

Uh, the patient is the bald guy laying in the bed with the chemo port hanging out of his body! Why is she asking this ridiculous question? Then she said, "well, this cannot be right. There is no way that you, Sir, have ovarian cancer."

Turns out that "Cruz" was a first name and the woman named Cruz with ovarian cancer had not heard them call out "Cruz". What I will never understand is why that first nurse looked at his ID and took his vitals, never noticing he was a man whose ID didn't match her chart. Thankfully, Bill didn't end up doing chemo for ovarian cancer that night.

Also, a lot of folks might get angry about this mess up. But no harm was done. To us, it was just another funny story and another great laugh.

I was used to hearing nurses walk out and call for Bill with all kinds of interesting pronunciations, but this was was my favorite! This nurse walks out and calls, "J.R." Bill got up to go with her and I looked at him like he was crazy. "What are you doing," I asked, "she didn't call you. She called for someone named J.R."

"I'll explain in a minute," he replied as he went with the nurse to get his weight and blood pressure. When he returned, I asked how he knew that "J.R." meant him. Well, you see, Bill's full name is William Wayne Crews, Jr. Yes, he is a junior and she had just looked at the "Jr" part and called him "JR"!!!! We loved this name so much that I still sometimes call him that. 🤣

your turn!

write some top tens together so you'll always have a good laugh

TOP TEN_____

TOP TEN_____

TUMOR HUMOR

funny →

How many cancer patients does it take to change a light bulb?

None. They are all to weak to climb the ladder.

Laughter is good medicine!

I'll share a few jokes we have heard over the years on these next pages and then give you some space to write out some you have heard or to make up your own!

Humor helps more than you can imagine! No, cancer is absolutely not funny. It is an evil, hideous monster that I hate more than words can describe. But I refused then and now to let cancer take away my sense of humor. I laughed at it as a weapon. If you find tumor humor offensive, skip the next few pages, but if you laugh like we did, I hope you enjoy this section of the book!

Knock Knock
Who's There?
The Interrupting Doctor.
The Interrupting Doc...
"You have cancer"!

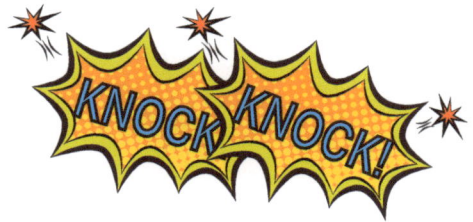

Knock Knock
Who's There?
Hugh
Hugh who?
Hugh look like crap!

Knock Knock
Who's There?
Boo
Boo who?
Don't cry. It's just cancer!

Knock Knock
Who's There?
Cancer.
Cancer who?
Knock Knock
Who's There?
Cancer.
Cancer who?
Knock Knock
Who's There?
Cancer.
Cancer who?
Knock Knock
Who's There?
Orange.
Orange who?
Orange you glad I didn't say CANCER?

Knock Knock
Who's There?
Watt.
Watt who?
Watt happened to your hair?

Knock Knock
Who's There?
Cancer.
Go away.

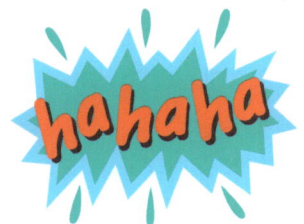

WARNING: These might be offensive!

What did the blonde do when she learned that 1 in 8 women get breast cancer?
She decided to hang out in groups of 7 or fewer.

Everyone tells you that smoking causes cancer. What they don't tell you is that it cures salmon.

I've heard like 7 cancer jokes today. If I hear "tumor", it's gonna benign.

I don't know why people say cancer is so hard to beat. I'm already on stage 4.

Why did the cancer specialist keep getting calls all night long? He was an on-call-ogist.

What do you call someone who keeps on getting lymphoma? A lymphomaniac!

I heard that 3 out of 5 people suffer from cancer. I guess the other 2 enjoy it.

Working together, write down some jokes you have heard to make you laugh through the pain.
Or... make up your own!

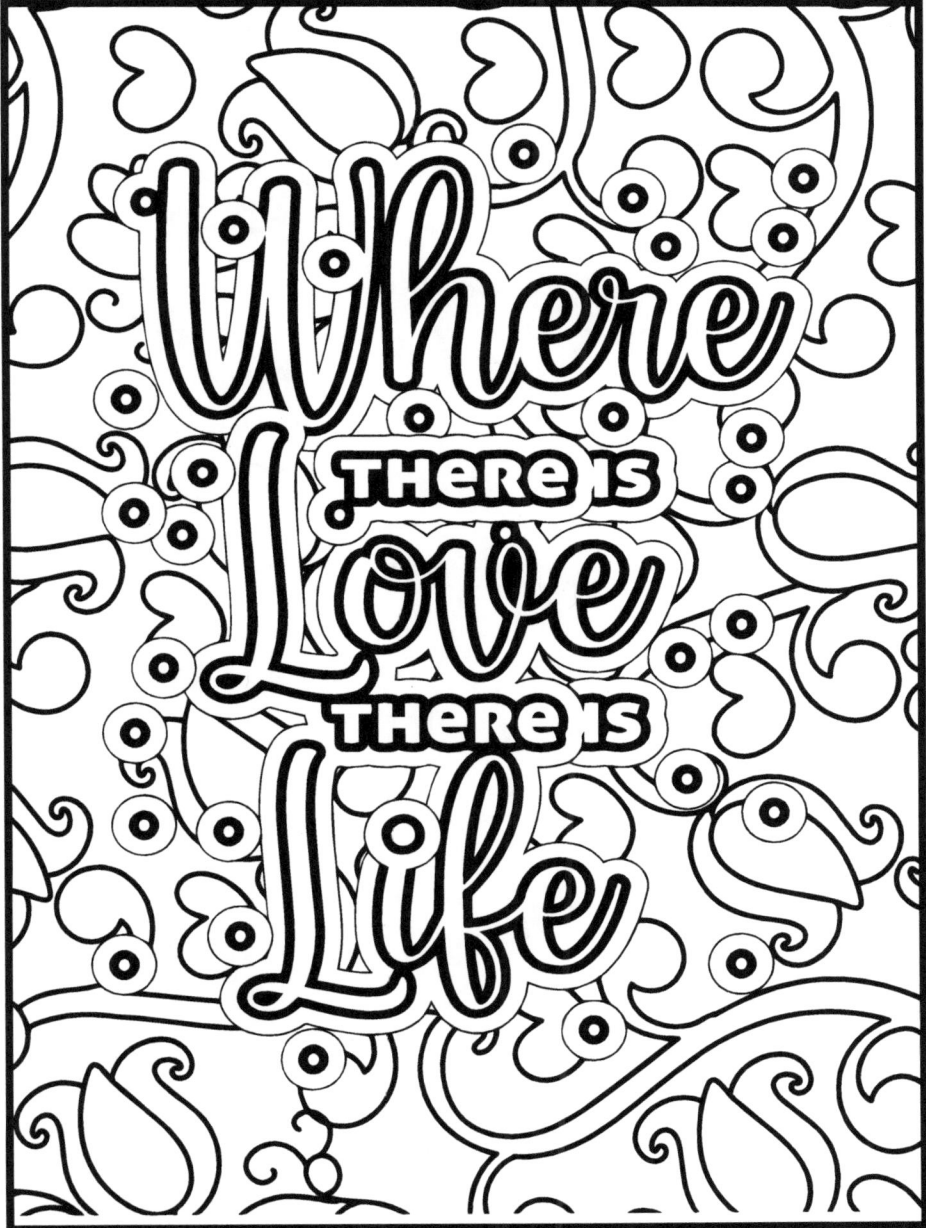

Where THERE IS Love THERE IS Life

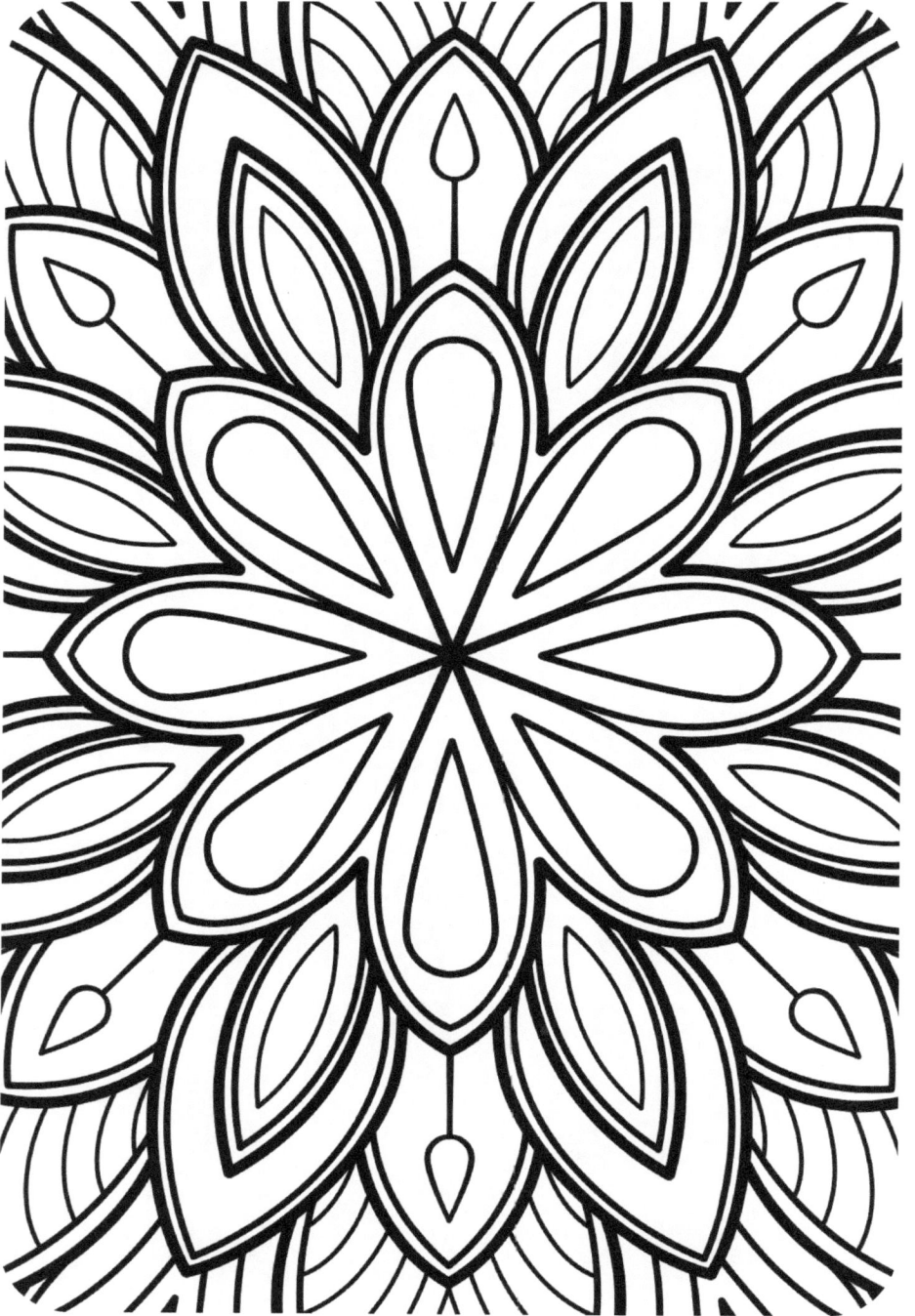

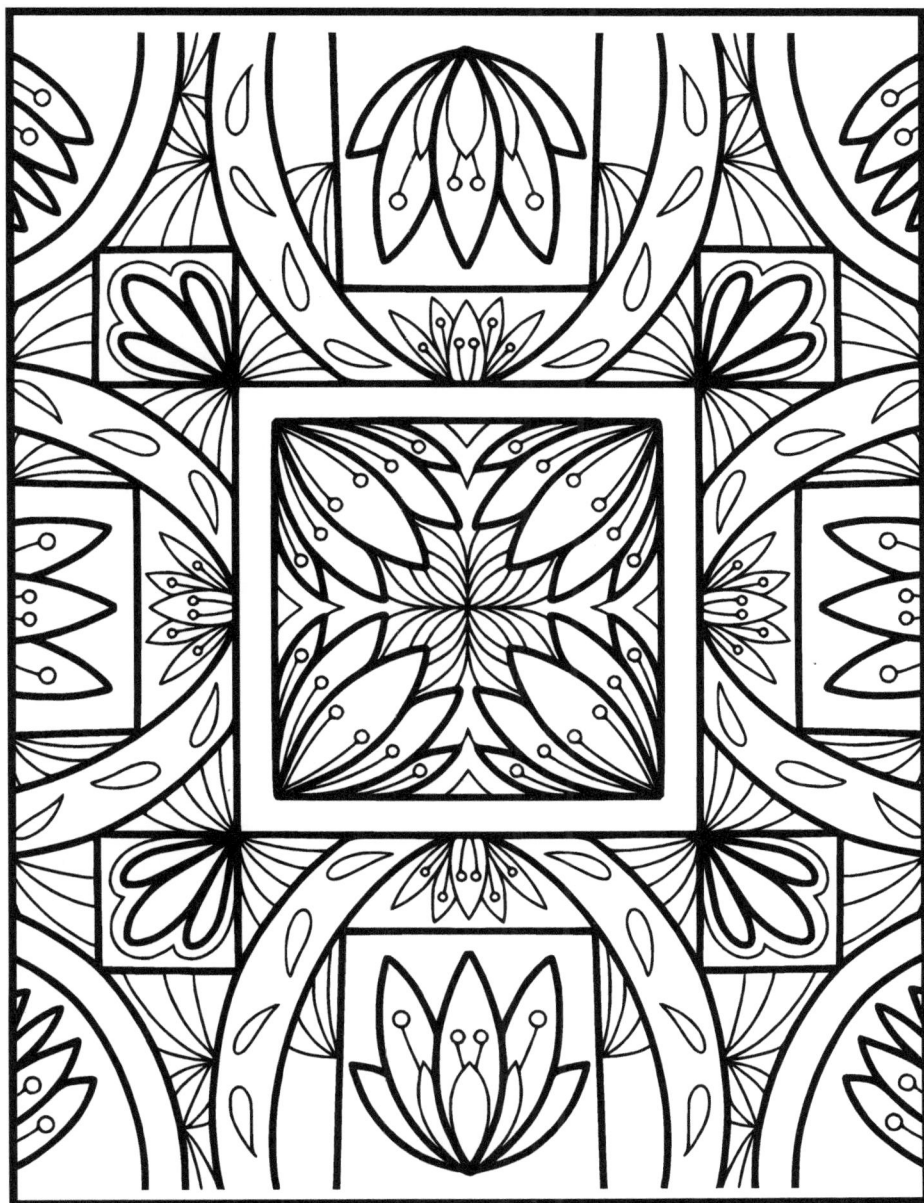

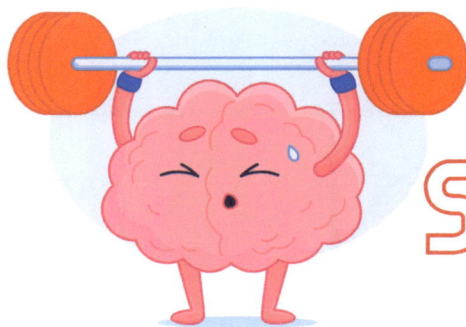

BRAIN STRENGTH

Use these brain teasers to help fight chemo brain (these are ones we saw/heard over the years of treatments)

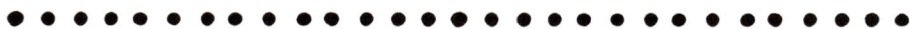

• •

A physician and a pilot were competing for the affections of a beautiful woman. The pilot was about to leave for a trip that would last for a week, so before he left, he gave the woman seven apples. Why?

There is a word in the English language in which the first two letters signify a male, the first three letters signify a female, the first four signify a great man, and the whole word, a great woman. What is the word?

What can be swallowed, but can also swallow you?

What is so unique about the number 8,549,176,320?

What is unusual about the following words: revive, banana, grammar, voodoo, assess, potato, dresser, uneven?

Is the capital of Kentucky pronounced Luis-ville or Luee-ville?

What can you hold in your left hand but not in your right?

What is 3/7 chicken, 2/3 cat and 2/4 goat?

I am heavy and impossible for you to pick up, but backwards I am not. What am I?

84% of people reading this will not find the the mistake in this

What occurs once in every minute, twice in every moment, yet never in a thousand years?

What is greater than God, more evil than the devil, the poor have it, the rich need it, and if you eat it, you'll die?

How do eight eights add up to 1,000?

What common English verb becomes its own past tense by rearranging its letters?

ANSWER KEY

A physician and a pilot were competing for the affections of a beautiful woman. The pilot was about to leave for a trip that would last for a week, so before he left, he gave the woman seven apples. Why?
An apple a day keeps the doctor away.

There is a word in the English language in which the first two letters signify a male, the first three letters signify a female, the first four signify a great man, and the whole word, a great woman. What is the word?
Heroine

What can be swallowed, but can also swallow you?
Pride

What is so unique about the number 8,549,176,320?
This is the only number that includes all of the digits in alphabetical order.

What is unusual about the following words: revive, banana, grammar, voodoo, assess, potato, dresser, uneven?
Take the first letter of each word and place it at the end. It will spell the same word backward.

Is the capital of Kentucky pronounced Luis-ville or Luee-ville?
Neither. The capital is Frankfurt.

What can you hold in your left hand but not in your right?
Your elbow.

What is 3/7 chicken, 2/3 cat and 2/4 goat?
Chicago

I am heavy and impossible for you to pick up, but backwards I am not. What am I?
Ton.

84% of people reading this will not find the the mistake in this
"the" is written twice

What occurs once in every minute, twice in every moment, yet never in a thousand years?
The letter "M"

What is greater than God, more evil than the devil, the poor have it, the rich need it, and if you eat it, you'll die?
Nothing.

How do eight eights add up to 1,000?
888 + 88 + 8 + 8 + 8 = 1000

What common English verb becomes its own past tense by rearranging its letters?
Eat (ate)

STUFF to do

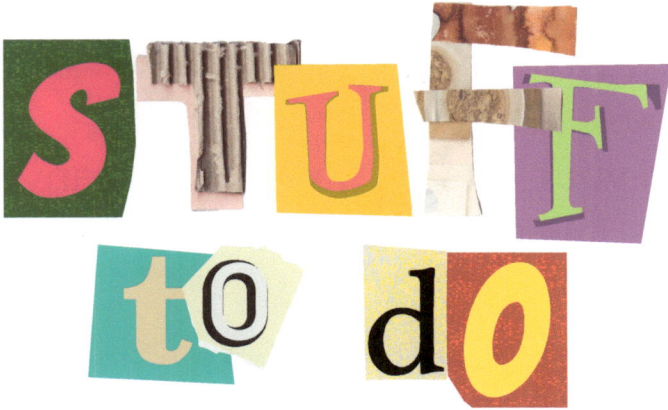

besides watching television

OK, you are home and you are both exhausted. You don't feel like watching television. What are some other ways to spend your time that both of you can do together?

slow dance in the kitchen

arts & crafts

read to each other

listen to music while holding hands

bake some cookies

buy a canvas and some paint and create a masterpiece

plan a trip for when you're better

write your story together

play a card game

have an indoor picnic

ACTIVITY: Write a list of 100 reasons you love your spouse. Both of you write a list and then read your lists out loud. How many are the same? How many surprised you?

ACTIVITY: Write a story together. Write about how you met and fell in love. Or write about some interesting adventures you've had together. Or maybe write about this time of illness and how you are trying to manage it. Maybe some day you can publish your story or hand it down to your children.

ACTIVITY: Have a family photo turned into a 500-piece puzzle and put it together while you enjoy your snacks.

ACTIVITY: Video yourselves slow dancing.

ACTIVITY: Look up some fun recipes and when you feel up to it, cook together.

ACTIVITY: Do a spa night. Do face masks and sugar scrubs and pedicures. Massage each other.

ACTIVITY: Make a fun time capsule together. Add photos and notes and special mementos from your relationship and bury it in the yard or hide it away somewhere. Ten or twenty years from now, you will really enjoy digging it up and remembering.

ACTIVITY: Have a pajama party. Make pancakes for dinner and put blankets and pillows on the floor. Relax and talk about unimportant things for a bit or just watch a funny movie.

ACTIVITY: Paint party. Sip some wine (or grape juice if that chemo patient can't have wine) while you paint a masterpiece on canvas. Or, maybe you want a new accent wall in your bedroom. As long as the patient has the strength, paint together!

ACTIVITY: Tour a museum right from your bed. Today, many museums offer virtual tours so you can go anywhere in the world.

ACTIVITY: Speaking of going anywhere, there are some really cool live feeds from different places that you can just sit and watch. One that is sometimes fascinating is Times Square. You can just sit and people watch and pretend you're hanging out in New York City.

ACTIVITY: Speaking of New York City, why not stream a broadway musical together? And if you both feel up to it, get all dressed up and pretend you're really there. Take cool photos of the evening (these can go in your time capsule).

ACTIVITY: Watch a sporting event together. Do you both like hockey? Put on your jersey and grab your snacks and cheer loud and proud for your team just like you're actually there.

ACTIVITY: Escape Room! There are some online kits you can buy or you can create your very own escape room and have a bit of fun trying to get out.

ACTIVITY: Picnic in the mountains or at the beach or in a beautiful field filled with flowers all from the comfort of home or even the hospital room. You see, you can find hours of either live feeds or pre-recorded loops of beautiful places. Just use your imagination and pretending to be there will soon feel like you really are there for a bit. Enjoy your meal together from anywhere you choose.

ACTIVITY: Join a virtual Pilates or Yoga class. These exercises are actually really good for that chemo patient and the caregiver needs it just as much. Grab a mat, y'all.

ACTIVITY: Find a good book and real out loud to each other.

ACTIVITY: Make S'mores in the fire pit. Wrap up in blankets and tell stories.

ACTIVITY: Imagine. Tell each other what you would be doing if only you could. Write it down and maybe, someday you can actually do it.

I am Not expert oN Relationships. I am No expert oN caNceR aNd chemo. I am just someoNe who has had to get cReative through sickNess aNd I have leaRNed that choosiNg love is always a good choice. LoviNg my husbaNd iN health is way easieR, but loviNg him iN sickNess, I have discoveRed is way moRe pRofouNd. Choose Love, y'all aNd go eNjoy youR Next Chemo Date.